MITCHELL BITNER

Calisthenics For You

Fortifying Natural Body Mechanics to Conquer Everyday Life!

First edition

This book was professionally typeset on Reedsy.
Find out more at reedsy.com

"It's not the destination, it's the journey"

Ralph Waldo Emerson

Contents

1	Introduction	1
2	What's Inside	2
3	My Fitness Background	3
4	The Recipe for Success	5
5	Planning Rest Days	6
6	Muscle Groups & Body Mechanics	7
7	Disclaimer	8
8	WOD 1	9
9	WOD 2	11
10	WOD 3	13
11	WOD 4	15
12	WOD 5	17
13	WOD 6	19
14	WOD 7	21
15	WOD 8	23
16	WOD 9	25
17	WOD 10	27
18	WOD 11	29
19	WOD 12	31
20	WOD 13	33
21	WOD 14	35
22	WOD 15 - Halfway through, you're doing awesome!	37
23	WOD 16	39
24	WOD 17	41

25	WOD 18	43
26	WOD 19	45
27	WOD 20	47
28	WOD 21	49
29	WOD 22	51
30	WOD 23	53
31	WOD 24	55
32	WOD 25	57
33	WOD 26	59
34	WOD 27	61
35	WOD 28	63
36	WOD 29	65
37	WOD 30	67
38	Conclusion	69
39	References	70

1

Introduction

First and foremost, CONGRATULATIONS on summoning the will power deep within to take this bold step in making a life changing experience for yourself! If this workout guide is for a friend or loved one, you've just purchased a gift to last a lifetime and potentially start a new beginning for them! These workouts are for all ages to enjoy and benefit from. Last, but not least, ARE YOU READY TO CHANGE YOUR LIFE?!

Sign and date here _________________________________. This is a pact to yourself, that you will hold yourself accountable and take these steps for a stronger, healthier, more structurally sound and mentally fortified you!

2

What's Inside

This fitness guide is devised of 30 different body sculpting workouts lasting anywhere from 30 minutes to an hour! It will provide daily calisthenics, combined with hints of functional fitness workouts to follow, ultimately ingraining superior body mechanics to last a lifetime. Each WOD, "workout of the day," will start and conclude with stretching to help prevent injury. These workouts are bodyweight based and require minimal to even no equipment depending on your current fitness level. Don't be afraid to scale certain movements up or down to accommodate yourself. These exercises are meant to help build a strong foundation.

3

My Fitness Background

My fitness journey started where most have, as a kid, all the way through middle school, highschool, college, to where I am now. I participated in many sports and physical activities including, baseball, track and field, cross country, wrestling, football, volleyball, BMX, cycling, snowboarding, hockey, spartan races, obstacle courses, half marathons, olympic weightlifting, traditional weightlifting, crossfit, functional fitness, calisthenics, mma, boxing, jujitsu, motocross and motorcycle road racing. There's probably a few activities I missed, but point being, they're all great in their own way and have helped develop the man I am today.

After graduating college I continued to lift weights at a regular gym, simply to stay in shape and build muscle. One day leaving that gym, I stumbled upon a crossfit gym, that just so happened to be next store and I let curiosity peak my interest. Long story short, it was the beginning of my fitness journey I never knew I needed, but always wanted! Yes, it was intimidating at first, like anything for the first time, but it unlocked a new way of using my body as a whole to move weight and in simplest terms live life functionally. For about three to four years I excelled in competitions. I later realized, I can't compete forever. The human body just can't sustain that intensity forever. That's when functional fitness and calisthenics became a pathway I knew I could follow for the rest of my life, no matter how old I get. Calisthenics develop strength and flexibility by only using your body weight. Functional fitness is the building block for anything you do in life, like picking something up off the ground, carrying heavy objects, or putting something on a shelf. The combination of functional fitness and calisthenics is the yin & yang to living a long, strong, and healthy lifestyle. The combination of these two styles of fitness will create a synchronized and structurally sound body, no matter what age you are. These skills will strengthen your body mechanics from the inside out and help prevent the unnecessary wear and tear life has to offer.

When you boil it down, structurally sound body mechanics are the basis for anything you do in your daily life. You don't have to lift weights or become a bodybuilder to live a functional sound, physically fit life. Adding weight to an exercise is an option or the next level after calisthenics and functional fitness are instilled. It's like taking a math test, but you only studied for history or competing in a marathon and only bodybuilding. Remember that gravity is a constant. Gravity is the one variable constantly working against us. Don't let gravity ruin your body. Calisthenics and functional fitness are the key ingredients for longevity against gravity. You'll build dense, lean muscle, become naturally flexible, and develop body mechanics you'll use the rest of your life.

4

The Recipe for Success

Working out is one piece to the puzzle. Constituting a healthy diet, keeping yourself accountable, knowing why you're doing this, and setting goals is just as important as the training itself. Mindset is the one thing that makes or breaks habits. Humans are naturally habitual. Willing yourself to create this perfect storm all starts with one day. That one day turns into two days, that turns into three days, and so on and so forth. After manipulating your mind with successful behavior, and creating these good habits, you won't even know who you were before. The only thing you'll be concerned with is making each day you wake up better than the last. Always remember where you started, stay humble and do it for the betterment of yourself. That kind of aura created is so contagious, you'll be inspiring others and not even knowing it. Be an inspiration, be a leader, be the light people didn't know they needed. Who knows, you may have not only transformed your life, but the life of someone else's in the process!

5

Planning Rest Days

These workouts can be done back-to-back days, but rest is needed for proper muscle recovery. Having rest days or active recovery days is important. These can occur once every two or three days based on how you feel. Example being, you workout Monday, Tuesday, Wednesday, rest Thursday, workout Friday, Saturday, rest Sunday and repeat. Another example, you workout Monday, Tuesday, rest Wednesday, workout Thursday, Friday, Saturday, rest day Sunday and repeat. However you'd like to split your days up to fit your schedule is perfectly fine. You can progressively push yourself harder as you get stronger and challenge yourself more. Two or three rest days per week is recommended and those rest days can be active rest days. Active rest days typically include walking, hiking, chores around the house, or basically anything to get your heart rate up. This keeps your body in motion in between workout days to help stay motivated!

6

Muscle Groups & Body Mechanics

The muscles involved are chest, shoulders, hamstrings, back, calves, abdominals, arms, biceps, gluteals, legs, trapezius, latissimus dorsi, triceps, back, forearms, quadriceps, teres muscle, deltoids, and erector spinae.

Body mechanics consist of standing, sitting, carrying, holding, bending, and sleeping. There are four components that go along with body mechanics: good posture, muscle-groups, center of gravity / base support, and proper lifting technique. There are 7 movement patterns that calisthenics cover (Upper Push + Pull, Lower Push + Pull, Squat, Gait and Rotation).

Functional movements are focussing groups of muscles together and moving them in synchronization. There are multiple joints of motion while performing functional fitness. These lifts transpire into everyday life, like walking, bending to pick something up, or moving heavy objects from the floor to higher locations.

Disclaimer

The publisher and the author strongly recommend that you consult with your physician before beginning any exercise program. You should be in good physical condition and be able to participate in the exercise. The author is not a licensed healthcare care provider and represents that they have no expertise in diagnosing, examining, or treating medical conditions of any kind, or in determining the effect of any specific exercise on a medical condition.

You should understand that when participating in any exercise or exercise program, there is the possibility of physical injury. If you engage in this exercise or exercise program, you agree that you do so at your own risk, are voluntarily participating in these activities, assume all risk of injury to yourself, and agree to release and discharge the publisher and the author from any and all claims or causes of action, known or unknown, arising out of the contents of this book.

The publisher and the author advise you to take full responsibility for your safety and know your limits. Before practicing the skills described in this book, be sure that your equipment is well maintained and do not take risks beyond your level of experience, aptitude, training, and comfort level.

WOD 1

Warm-up:

A light, dynamic warm-up complimenting each movement is recommended. Examples: leg swings, arm circles, torso twists and other dynamic movements to prepare your muscles and joints.

Perform each exercise in order for 3-4 rounds. Rest for 30-60 seconds between each exercise.

Workout:
1. Push-Ups (10-15 reps)
2. Bodyweight Squats (15 reps)
3. Pull-Ups or Inverted Rows (8-12 reps)
4. Lunges (12 reps per leg)
5. Dips (10-15 reps)
6. Plank (30-60 seconds)
7. Mountain Climbers (20 reps)

Stretches:

1. Seated Forward Bend (2 minutes): Stretch the hamstrings and lower back.

2. Child's Pose (1 minute): Relax and stretch the lower back and hips.

3. Triceps Stretch (1 minute per arm): Stretch the triceps to relieve tension.

4. Cobra Stretch (1 minute): Open up the chest and stretch the abdominal muscles.

5. Quad Stretch (1 minute per leg): Stretch the front of the thighs.

9

WOD 2

Warm-up:

A light, dynamic warm-up complimenting each movement is recommended. Examples: leg swings, arm circles, torso twists and other dynamic movements to prepare your muscles and joints.

Perform each exercise in order for 3-4 rounds. Rest for 30-60 seconds between each exercise.

Workout:
1. Burpees (12 reps)
2. Lunges with a Twist (12 reps per leg)
3. Toes-To-Bar (12-15 reps)
4. Bodyweight Rows (12 reps)
5. Bodyweight Squats (15 reps)
6. Plank to Alternating Toe Touch (15 reps)
7. Double Unders (30 reps) or Single Unders (60 reps)

Stretches:

1. Seated Forward Fold (2 minutes): Stretch the hamstrings and lower back.

2. Chest Opener Stretch (1 minute): Open up the chest and shoulders.

3. Hip Flexor Stretch (1 minute per leg): Release tension in the hips and thighs.

4. Child's Pose (1 minute): Relax and stretch the lower back and hips.

5. Triceps Stretch (1 minute per arm): Stretch the triceps to relieve tension.

10

WOD 3

Warm-up:

A light, dynamic warm-up complimenting each movement is recommended. Examples: leg swings, arm circles, torso twists and other dynamic movements to prepare your muscles and joints.

Perform each exercise in order for 3-4 rounds. Rest for 30-60 seconds between each exercise.

Workout:
1. Skater Jumps (10 reps per leg)
2. Push-Ups (12-15 reps)
3. Walking Lunges (20 steps)
4. Handstand Push-Ups (8-10 reps)
5. Plank to Tuck Jump (12 reps)
6. Box Jumps (15 reps) "Height of box jump is personal preference"
7. Hanging Leg Raises (12 reps)

Stretches:

1. Seated Forward Bend (2 minutes): Stretch the hamstrings and lower back.

2. Cobra Stretch (1 minute): Open up the chest and stretch the abdominal muscles.

3. Quad Stretch (1 minute per leg): Stretch the front of the thighs.

4. Triceps Stretch (1 minute per arm): Stretch the triceps to relieve tension.

5. Child's Pose (2 minutes): Relax and stretch the lower back, hips, and shoulders.

11

WOD 4

Warm-up:

A light, dynamic warm-up complimenting each movement is recommended. Examples: leg swings, arm circles, torso twists and other dynamic movements to prepare your muscles and joints.

Perform each exercise in order for 3-4 rounds. Rest for 30-60 seconds between each exercise.

Workout:
1. Handstand Push-Ups (8-10 reps)
2. Bodyweight Squats (15 reps)
3. Dips (15 reps)
4. Lunges with a Twist (12 reps per leg)
5. Hollow Body Hold (hold for 30 seconds)
6. Mountain Climbers (20 reps per side)
7. Box or Bench Step-Ups (15 reps per leg)

Stretches:

1. Seated Forward Bend (2 minutes): Stretch the hamstrings and lower back.

2. Chest Opener Stretch (1 minute): Open up the chest and shoulders.

3. Hip Flexor Stretch (1 minute per leg): Release tension in the hips and thighs.

4. Triceps Stretch (1 minute per arm): Stretch the triceps to relieve tension.

5. Child's Pose (2 minutes): Relax and stretch the lower back, hips, and shoulders.

12

WOD 5

Warm-up:

A light, dynamic warm-up complimenting each movement is recommended. Examples: leg swings, arm circles, torso twists and other dynamic movements to prepare your muscles and joints.

Perform each exercise in order for 3-4 rounds. Rest for 30-60 seconds between each exercise.

Workout:
1. Hand Release Push-Ups (12-15 reps)
2. Bodyweight Squats (15 reps)
3. Australian Pull-Ups (12-15 reps)
4. Pike Push-Ups (12-15 reps)
5. Walking Lunges (20 steps)
6. Tuck Jumps (15 reps)
7. Plank to Side Plank (12 reps per side)

Stretches:

1. Seated Forward Bend (2 minutes): Stretch the hamstrings and lower back.

2. Child's Pose (1 minute): Relax and stretch the lower back, hips, and shoulders.

3. Doorway Chest Stretch (1 minute): Open up the chest and stretch the front of the shoulders.

4. Quad Stretch (1 minute per leg): Stretch the front of the thighs.

5. Triceps Stretch (1 minute per arm): Stretch the triceps to relieve tension.

13

WOD 6

Warm-up:

A light, dynamic warm-up complimenting each movement is recom-mended. Examples: leg swings, arm circles, torso twists and other dynamic movements to prepare your muscles and joints.

Perform each exercise in order for 3-4 rounds. Rest for 30-60 seconds between each exercise.

Workout:
1. Clapping Push-Ups (12 reps)
2. Squat Jumps (15 reps)
3. Bodyweight Rows on Rings or Bar (12 reps)
4. Commando Pull-Ups (10 reps)
5. Hanging Knee Raises (15 reps)
6. Side Lunges (12 reps per leg)
7. Plank to Pike (12 reps)

Stretches:

1. Forward Fold (2 minutes): Stretch the hamstrings and lower back.

2. Seated Twist (1 minute per side): Rotate your torso to stretch the spine and engage the obliques.

3. Hip Flexor Stretch (1 minute per leg): Stretch the front of the hips and thighs.

4. Cat-Cow Stretch (2 minutes): Mobilize the spine and stretch the back.

5. Calf Stretch (1 minute per leg): Stretch the calves for lower leg flexibility.

14

WOD 7

Warm-up:

A light, dynamic warm-up complimenting each movement is recommended. Examples: leg swings, arm circles, torso twists and other dynamic movements to prepare your muscles and joints.

Perform each exercise in order for 3-4 rounds. Rest for 30-60 seconds between each exercise.

Workout:
1. Explosive Push-Ups (12 reps)
2. Box Jumps (15 reps) "Height of box jump is personal preference"
3. L-Sit Pull-Ups (10 reps)
4. Plyometric Lunges (20 reps)
5. Body Rows on Rings (12 reps)
6. Tuck Planche Holds (hold for 20-30 seconds)
7. Handstand Wall Walks (5 walks)

Stretches:

1. Seated Forward Bend (2 minutes): Stretch the hamstrings and lower back.

2. Child's Pose (1 minute): Relax and stretch the lower back, hips, and shoulders.

3. Thoracic Spine Rotation (1 minute per side): Improve mobility in the upper back.

4. Quad Stretch (1 minute per leg): Stretch the front of the thighs.

5. Triceps Stretch (1 minute per arm): Stretch the triceps to relieve tension.

15

WOD 8

Warm-up:

A light, dynamic warm-up complimenting each movement is recommended. Examples: leg swings, arm circles, torso twists and other dynamic movements to prepare your muscles and joints.

Perform each exercise in order for 3-4 rounds. Rest for 30-60 seconds between each exercise.

Workout:
1. One-Arm Push-Ups (8 reps per arm)
2. Box Pistols (8 reps per leg)
3. Wall Handstand (hold for 30 seconds)
4. Bodyweight Tricep Extensions (12 reps)
5. Bicycle Crunches (20 reps)
6. Plyometric Box Push-Ups (12 reps)
7. Single-Leg Glute Bridge (15 reps per leg)

Stretches:

1. Forward Fold (2 minutes): Stretch the hamstrings and lower back.

2. Seated Twist (1 minute per side): Rotate your torso to stretch the spine and engage the obliques.

3. Hip Flexor Stretch (1 minute per leg): Stretch the front of the hips and thighs.

4. Cat-Cow Stretch (2 minutes): Mobilize the spine and stretch the back.

5. Triceps Stretch (1 minute per arm): Stretch the triceps to relieve tension.

16

WOD 9

Warm-up:

A light, dynamic warm-up complimenting each movement is recommended. Examples: leg swings, arm circles, torso twists and other dynamic movements to prepare your muscles and joints.

Perform each exercise in order for 3-4 rounds. Rest for 30-60 seconds between each exercise.

Workout:
1. Explosive Burpees (12 reps)
2. Dragon Flags (4 sets of 8 reps)
3. Pistol Squats (10 reps per leg)
4. Wide Grip Pull-Ups (3 sets of 12 reps)
5. Plank to Side Plank with Leg Lift (12 reps per side)
6. Box Jumps (15 reps) "Height of box jump is personal preference"
7. Hanging Leg Raises (15 reps)

Stretches:

1. Seated Forward Bend (2 minutes): Stretch the hamstrings and lower back.

2. Child's Pose (1 minute): Relax and stretch the lower back, hips, and shoulders.

3. Chest Opener Stretch (1 minute): Open up the chest and stretch the shoulders.

4. Quad Stretch (1 minute per leg): Stretch the front of the thighs.

5. Triceps Stretch (1 minute per arm): Stretch the triceps to relieve tension.

WOD 10

Warm-up:

A light, dynamic warm-up complimenting each movement is recommended. Examples: leg swings, arm circles, torso twists and other dynamic movements to prepare your muscles and joints.

Perform each exercise in order for 3-4 rounds. Rest for 30-60 seconds between each exercise.

Workout:
1. Diamond Push-Ups (12 reps)
2. Jumping Lunges (20 reps)
3. Pull-Ups with Leg Raises (10 reps)
4. Box Pistols (10 reps per leg)
5. Dips between Parallel Bars (15 reps)
6. L-Sit (hold for 20 seconds)
7. Hanging Windshield Wipers (12 reps per side)

Stretches:

1. Seated Forward Bend (2 minutes): Stretch the hamstrings and lower back.

2. Child's Pose (1 minute): Relax and stretch the lower back, hips, and shoulders.

3. Thoracic Spine Rotation (1 minute per side): Improve mobility in the upper back.

4. Quad Stretch (1 minute per leg): Stretch the front of the thighs.

5. Triceps Stretch (1 minute per arm): Stretch the triceps to relieve tension.

18

WOD 11

Warm-up:

A light, dynamic warm-up complimenting each movement is recommended. Examples: leg swings, arm circles, torso twists and other dynamic movements to prepare your muscles and joints.

Perform each exercise in order for 3-4 rounds. Rest for 30-60 seconds between each exercise.

Workout:
1. Explosive Push-Ups (4 sets of 12 reps)
2. Jumping Jacks (20 reps)
3. Wide Grip Pull-Ups (10 reps)
4. Box Jumps (15 reps) "Height of box jump is personal preference"
5. Hanging Leg Raises (15 reps)
6. Archer Rows (12 reps per arm)
7. Dips (15 reps)

Stretches:

1. Seated Forward Bend (2 minutes): Stretch the hamstrings and lower back.

2. Child's Pose (1 minute): Relax and stretch the lower back, hips, and shoulders.

3. Thoracic Spine Rotation (1 minute per side): Improve mobility in the upper back.

4. Quad Stretch (1 minute per leg): Stretch the front of the thighs.

5. Triceps Stretch (1 minute per arm): Stretch the triceps to relieve tension.

WOD 12

Warm-up:

A light, dynamic warm-up complimenting each movement is recommended. Examples: leg swings, arm circles, torso twists and other dynamic movements to prepare your muscles and joints.

Perform each exercise in order for 3-4 rounds. Rest for 30-60 seconds between each exercise.

Workout:
1. Planche Progression (hold for 20 seconds)
2. Bulgarian Split Squats (12 reps per leg)
3. Muscle-Ups (6 reps)
4. Tuck Jumps (15 reps)
5. Toes-To-Bar (12-15 reps)
6. Back Lever Progression (hold for 15 seconds)
7. Lateral Lunges (12 reps per leg)

Stretches:

1. Seated Forward Bend (2 minutes): Stretch the hamstrings and lower back.

2. Child's Pose (1 minute): Relax and stretch the lower back, hips, and shoulders.

3. Triceps Stretch (1 minute per arm): Stretch the triceps to relieve tension.

4. Cobra Stretch (1 minute): Open up the chest and stretch the abdominal muscles.

5. Quad Stretch (1 minute per leg): Stretch the front of the thighs.

20

WOD 13

Warm-up:

A light, dynamic warm-up complimenting each movement is recommended. Examples: leg swings, arm circles, torso twists and other dynamic movements to prepare your muscles and joints.

Perform each exercise in order for 3-4 rounds. Rest for 30-60 seconds between each exercise.

Workout:
1. Explosive Burpees (12 reps)
2. Cossack Squats (10 reps per leg)
3. Box Jumps (15 reps) "Height of box jump is personal preference"
4. Plank with Leg Raises (15 raises per leg)
5. Bicycle Crunches (20 reps)
6. Jumping Lunges (20 reps)
7. Triceps Dips (15 reps)

Stretches:

1. Seated Forward Bend (2 minutes): Stretch the hamstrings and lower back.

2. Child's Pose (1 minute): Relax and stretch the lower back, hips, and shoulders.

3. Chest Opener Stretch (1 minute): Open up the chest and stretch the shoulders.

4. Quad Stretch (1 minute per leg): Stretch the front of the thighs.

5. Triceps Stretch (1 minute per arm): Stretch the triceps to relieve tension.

21

WOD 14

Warm-up:

A light, dynamic warm-up complimenting each movement is recommended. Examples: leg swings, arm circles, torso twists and other dynamic movements to prepare your muscles and joints.

Perform each exercise in order for 3-4 rounds. Rest for 30-60 seconds between each exercise.

Workout:
1. One-Arm Push-Ups (8 reps per arm)
2. Jump Squats (15 reps)
3. Commando Pull-Ups (8-12 reps)
4. Lunges with Rotation (12 reps per leg)
5. Dragon Flags (10 reps)
6. Lateral Box Jumps (12 reps per side)
7. Hanging Windshield Wipers (12 reps per side)

Stretches:

1. Seated Forward Bend (2 minutes): Stretch the hamstrings and lower back.

2. Child's Pose (1 minute): Relax and stretch the lower back, hips, and shoulders.

3. Thoracic Spine Rotation (1 minute per side): Improve mobility in the upper back.

4. Quad Stretch (1 minute per leg): Stretch the front of the thighs.

5. Triceps Stretch (1 minute per arm): Stretch the triceps to relieve tension.

22

WOD 15 - Halfway through, you're doing awesome!

Warm-up:

A light, dynamic warm-up complimenting each movement is recommended. Examples: leg swings, arm circles, torso twists and other dynamic movements to prepare your muscles and joints.

Perform each exercise in order for 3-4 rounds. Rest for 30-60 seconds between each exercise.

Workout:
1. Handstand Push-Ups (8-10 reps)
2. L-Sit Pull-Ups (8-10 reps)
3. Pistol Squats (10 reps per leg)
4. Muscle-Ups (6 reps)
5. Hollow Body Hold (hold for 30 seconds)
6. Box Jumps (15 reps) "Height of box jump is personal preference"
7. Dips with Knee Tucks (12 reps)

Stretches:

1. Seated Forward Bend (2 minutes): Stretch the hamstrings and lower back.

2. Child's Pose (1 minute): Relax and stretch the lower back, hips, and shoulders.

3. Chest Opener Stretch (1 minute): Open up the chest and stretch the shoulders.

4. Quad Stretch (1 minute per leg): Stretch the front of the thighs.

5. Triceps Stretch (1 minute per arm): Stretch the triceps to relieve tension.

23

WOD 16

Warm-up:

A light, dynamic warm-up complimenting each movement is recommended. Examples: leg swings, arm circles, torso twists and other dynamic movements to prepare your muscles and joints.

Perform each exercise in order for 3-4 rounds. Rest for 30-60 seconds between each exercise.

Workout:
1. Clapping Pull-Ups (10 reps)
2. Jump Squats (15 reps)
3. Archer Push-Ups (12 reps)
4. Double Unders (30 reps) or Single Unders (60 reps)
5. Muscle-Ups (6 reps)
6. Plyometric Box Push-Ups (15 reps)
7. Tuck Jumps (15 reps)

Stretches:

1. Seated Forward Bend (2 minutes): Stretch the hamstrings and lower back.

2. Child's Pose (1 minute): Relax and stretch the lower back, hips, and shoulders.

3. Triceps Stretch (1 minute per arm): Stretch the triceps to relieve tension.

4. Chest Opener Stretch (1 minute): Open up the chest and stretch the shoulders.

5. Quad Stretch (1 minute per leg): Stretch the front of the thighs.

WOD 17

Warm-up:

A light, dynamic warm-up complimenting each movement is recommended. Examples: leg swings, arm circles, torso twists and other dynamic movements to prepare your muscles and joints.

Perform each exercise in order for 3-4 rounds. Rest for 30-60 seconds between each exercise.

Workout:
1. Planche Lean (hold for 20 seconds)
2. Box or Bench Step-Ups (15 reps per leg)
3. Wide Grip Pull-Ups (12 reps)
4. Box Pistols (10 reps per leg)
5. Handstand Push-Ups (12 reps)
6. Dips between Parallel Bars (15 reps)
7. Dragon Flags (10 reps)

Stretches:

1. Seated Forward Bend (2 minutes): Stretch the hamstrings and lower back.

2. Child's Pose (1 minute): Relax and stretch the lower back, hips, and shoulders.

3. Triceps Stretch (1 minute per arm): Stretch the triceps to relieve tension.

4. Chest Opener Stretch (1 minute): Open up the chest and stretch the shoulders.

5. Quad Stretch (1 minute per leg): Stretch the front of the thighs.

25

WOD 18

Warm-up:

A light, dynamic warm-up complimenting each movement is recommended. Examples: leg swings, arm circles, torso twists and other dynamic movements to prepare your muscles and joints.

Perform each exercise in order for 3-4 rounds. Rest for 30-60 seconds between each exercise.

Workout:
1. Clapping Push-Ups (12 reps)
2. Box Jumps (15 reps) "Height of box jump is personal preference"
3. L-Sit Pull-Ups (8 reps)
4. Jumping Jacks (20 reps)
5. Handstand Wall Holds (hold for 30 seconds)
6. Body Rows on Rings (12 reps)
7. Skater Jumps (10 per leg)

Stretches:

1. Seated Forward Bend (2 minutes): Stretch the hamstrings and lower back.

2. Child's Pose (1 minute): Relax and stretch the lower back, hips, and shoulders.

3. Triceps Stretch (1 minute per arm): Stretch the triceps to relieve tension.

4. Cobra Stretch (1 minute): Open up the chest and stretch the abdominal muscles.

5. Quad Stretch (1 minute per leg): Stretch the front of the thighs.

26

WOD 19

Warm-up:

A light, dynamic warm-up complimenting each movement is recommended. Examples: leg swings, arm circles, torso twists and other dynamic movements to prepare your muscles and joints.

Perform each exercise in order for 3-4 rounds. Rest for 30-60 seconds between each exercise.

Workout:
1. Explosive Pull-Ups (10 reps)
2. Bulgarian Split Squats (12 reps per leg)
3. L-Sit to Handstand (5 reps)
4. Box or Bench Step-Ups (15 reps per leg)
5. Bicycle Crunches (20 reps)
6. Jumping Lunges (20 reps)
7. Triceps Dips (15 reps)

Stretches:

1. Seated Forward Bend (2 minutes): Stretch the hamstrings and lower back.

2. Child's Pose (1 minute): Relax and stretch the lower back, hips, and shoulders.

3. Triceps Stretch (1 minute per arm): Stretch the triceps to relieve tension.

4. Chest Opener Stretch (1 minute): Open up the chest and stretch the shoulders.

5. Quad Stretch (1 minute per leg): Stretch the front of the thigh

27

WOD 20

Warm-up:

A light, dynamic warm-up complimenting each movement is recommended. Examples: leg swings, arm circles, torso twists and other dynamic movements to prepare your muscles and joints.

Perform each exercise in order for 3-4 rounds. Rest for 30-60 seconds between each exercise.

Workout:
1. Pistol Squats (8 reps per leg)
2. Wide Grip Pull-Ups (10 reps)
3. Broad Jumps (8-10 jumps)
4. Hanging Leg Raises (15 reps)
5. Archer Rows (12 reps per arm)
6. Handstand Practice (hold for 30 seconds)
7. Explosive Burpees (12 reps)

Stretches:

1. Seated Forward Bend (2 minutes): Stretch the hamstrings and lower back.

2. Child's Pose (1 minute): Relax and stretch the lower back, hips, and shoulders.

3. Triceps Stretch (1 minute per arm): Stretch the triceps to relieve tension.

4. Chest Opener Stretch (1 minute): Open up the chest and stretch the shoulders.

5. Quad Stretch (1 minute per leg): Stretch the front of the thighs.

WOD 21

Warm-up:

A light, dynamic warm-up complimenting each movement is recommended. Examples: leg swings, arm circles, torso twists and other dynamic movements to prepare your muscles and joints.

Perform each exercise in order for 3-4 rounds. Rest for 30-60 seconds between each exercise.

Workout:
1. Clapping Pull-Ups (10 reps)
2. Jump Squats (15 reps)
3. Archer Push-Ups (12 reps)
4. Cossack Squats (10 reps per leg)
5. Muscle-Ups (6 reps)
6. Plyometric Box Push-Ups (15 reps)
7. L-Sit (hold for 20 seconds)

Stretches:

1. Seated Forward Bend (2 minutes): Stretch the hamstrings and lower back.

2. Child's Pose (1 minute): Relax and stretch the lower back, hips, and shoulders.

3. Triceps Stretch (1 minute per arm): Stretch the triceps to relieve tension.

4. Chest Opener Stretch (1 minute): Open up the chest and stretch the shoulders.

5. Quad Stretch (1 minute per leg): Stretch the front of the thighs.

29

WOD 22

Warm-up:

A light, dynamic warm-up complimenting each movement is recommended. Examples: leg swings, arm circles, torso twists and other dynamic movements to prepare your muscles and joints.

Perform each exercise in order for 3-4 rounds. Rest for 30-60 seconds between each exercise.

Workout:
1. Explosive Burpees (12 reps)
2. Dragon Flags (8 reps)
3. L-Sit Pull-Ups (10 reps)
4. Bulgarian Split Squats (12 reps per leg)
5. Plank to Side Plank with Leg Lift (12 reps per side)
6. Box Jumps (15 reps) "Height of box jump is personal preference"
7. Dips with Knee Tucks (12 reps)

Stretches:

1. Seated Forward Bend (2 minutes): Stretch the hamstrings and lower back.

2. Child's Pose (1 minute): Relax and stretch the lower back, hips, and shoulders.

3. Chest Opener Stretch (1 minute): Open up the chest and stretch the shoulders.

4. Quad Stretch (1 minute per leg): Stretch the front of the thighs.

5. Triceps Stretch (1 minute per arm): Stretch the triceps to relieve tension.

30

WOD 23

Warm-up:

A light, dynamic warm-up complimenting each movement is recommended. Examples: leg swings, arm circles, torso twists and other dynamic movements to prepare your muscles and joints.

Perform each exercise in order for 3-4 rounds. Rest for 30-60 seconds between each exercise.

Workout:
1. Explosive Push-Ups (15 reps)
2. Pistol Squats (10 reps per leg)
3. Wide Grip Pull-Ups (12 reps)
4. Broad Jumps (8-10 jumps)
5. Tuck Planche Holds (hold for 20 seconds)
6. Hanging Windshield Wipers (12 reps per side)
7. Clapping Lunges (20 reps)

Stretches:

1. Seated Forward Bend (2 minutes): Stretch the hamstrings and lower back.

2. Child's Pose (1 minute): Relax and stretch the lower back, hips, and shoulders.

3. Triceps Stretch (1 minute per arm): Stretch the triceps to relieve tension.

4. Cobra Stretch (1 minute): Open up the chest and stretch the abdominal muscles.

5. Quad Stretch (1 minute per leg): Stretch the front of the thighs.

WOD 24

Warm-up:

A light, dynamic warm-up complimenting each movement is recommended. Examples: leg swings, arm circles, torso twists and other dynamic movements to prepare your muscles and joints.

Perform each exercise in order for 3-4 rounds. Rest for 30-60 seconds between each exercise.

Workout:
1. Clapping Pull-Ups (10 reps)
2. Jump Squats (15 reps)
3. One-Arm Push-Ups (8 reps per arm)
4. Hanging Leg Raises (15 reps)
5. Handstand Wall Holds (hold for 30 seconds)
6. Skater Jumps (10 per leg)
7. Plyometric Box Push-Ups (15 reps)

Stretches:

1. Seated Forward Bend (2 minutes): Stretch the hamstrings and lower back.

2. Child's Pose (1 minute): Relax and stretch the lower back, hips, and shoulders.

3. Triceps Stretch (1 minute per arm): Stretch the triceps to relieve tension.

4. Chest Opener Stretch (1 minute): Open up the chest and stretch the shoulders.

5. Quad Stretch (1 minute per leg): Stretch the front of the thighs.

32

WOD 25

Warm-up:

A light, dynamic warm-up complimenting each movement is recommended. Examples: leg swings, arm circles, torso twists and other dynamic movements to prepare your muscles and joints.

Perform each exercise in order for 3-4 rounds. Rest for 30-60 seconds between each exercise.

Workout:
1. Explosive Push-Ups (15 reps)
2. Wide Grip Pull-Ups (12 reps)
3. Box Jumps (15 reps) "Height of box jump is personal preference"
4. L-Sit to Handstand Progression (5 reps)
5. Dips between Parallel Bars (15 reps)
6. Hanging Windshield Wipers (12 reps per side)
7. Clapping Lunges (20 reps)

Stretches:

1. Seated Forward Bend (2 minutes): Stretch the hamstrings and lower back.

2. Child's Pose (1 minute): Relax and stretch the lower back, hips, and shoulders.

3. Triceps Stretch (1 minute per arm): Stretch the triceps to relieve tension.

4. Cobra Stretch (1 minute): Open up the chest and stretch the abdominal muscles.

5. Quad Stretch (1 minute per leg): Stretch the front of the thighs.

33

WOD 26

Warm-up:

A light, dynamic warm-up complimenting each movement is recommended. Examples: leg swings, arm circles, torso twists and other dynamic movements to prepare your muscles and joints.

Perform each exercise in order for 3-4 rounds. Rest for 30-60 seconds between each exercise.

Workout:
1. Commando Pull-Ups (8-12 reps)
2. Jump Squats (15 reps)
3. Archer Push-Ups (12 reps)
4. Jumping Jacks (20 reps)
5. Bulgarian Split Squats (12 reps per leg)
6. Hanging Leg Raises (15 reps)
7. Muscle-Ups (6 reps)

Stretches:

1. Seated Forward Bend (2 minutes): Stretch the hamstrings and lower back.

2. Child's Pose (1 minute): Relax and stretch the lower back, hips, and shoulders.

3. Triceps Stretch (1 minute per arm): Stretch the triceps to relieve tension.

4. Chest Opener Stretch (1 minute): Open up the chest and stretch the shoulders.

5. Quad Stretch (1 minute per leg): Stretch the front of the thighs.

34

WOD 27

Warm-up:

A light, dynamic warm-up complimenting each movement is recommended. Examples: leg swings, arm circles, torso twists and other
dynamic movements to prepare your muscles and joints.

Perform each exercise in order for 3-4 rounds. Rest for 30-60 seconds
between each exercise.

Workout:
1. Box or Bench Step-Ups (15 reps per leg)
2. Wide Grip Pull-Ups (12 reps)
3. Box Jumps (15 reps) "Height of box jump is personal preference"
4. Tuck Planche Holds (hold for 20 seconds)
5. Dips between Parallel Bars (15 reps)
6. Hanging Windshield Wipers (12 reps per side)
7. Clapping Lunges (20 reps)

Stretches:

1. Seated Forward Bend (2 minutes): Stretch the hamstrings and lower back.

2. Child's Pose (1 minute): Relax and stretch the lower back, hips, and shoulders.

3. Triceps Stretch (1 minute per arm): Stretch the triceps to relieve tension.

4. Cobra Stretch (1 minute): Open up the chest and stretch the abdominal muscles.

5. Quad Stretch (1 minute per leg): Stretch the front of the thighs.

35

WOD 28

Warm-up:

A light, dynamic warm-up complimenting each movement is recommended. Examples: leg swings, arm circles, torso twists and other dynamic movements to prepare your muscles and joints.

Perform each exercise in order for 3-4 rounds. Rest for 30-60 seconds between each exercise.

Workout:
1. Clapping Pull-Ups (10 reps)
2. Cossack Squats (10 reps per leg)
3. Hanging Leg Raises (15 reps)
4. Handstand Wall Holds (hold for 30 seconds)
5. One-Arm Push-Ups (8 reps per arm)
6. Plyometric Box Push-Ups (15 reps)
7. L-Sit (hold for 20 seconds)

Stretches:

1. Seated Forward Bend (2 minutes): Stretch the hamstrings and lower back.

2. Child's Pose (1 minute): Relax and stretch the lower back, hips, and shoulders.

3. Triceps Stretch (1 minute per arm): Stretch the triceps to relieve tension.

4. Chest Opener Stretch (1 minute): Open up the chest and stretch the shoulders.

5. Quad Stretch (1 minute per leg): Stretch the front of the thighs.

36

WOD 29

Warm-up:

A light, dynamic warm-up complimenting each movement is recommended. Examples: leg swings, arm circles, torso twists and other dynamic movements to prepare your muscles and joints.

Perform each exercise in order for 3-4 rounds. Rest for 30-60 seconds between each exercise.

Workout:
1. Diamond Push-Ups (12 reps)
2. Bulgarian Split Squats (12 reps per leg)
3. Wide Grip Pull-Ups (12 reps)
4. Box Jumps (15 reps) "Height of box jump is personal preference"
5. L-Sit to Handstand Progression (5 reps)
6. Dips between Parallel Bars (15 reps)
7. Clapping Lunges (20 reps)

Stretches:

1. Seated Forward Bend (2 minutes): Stretch the hamstrings and lower back.

2. Child's Pose (1 minute): Relax and stretch the lower back, hips, and shoulders.

3. Triceps Stretch (1 minute per arm): Stretch the triceps to relieve tension.

4. Cobra Stretch (1 minute): Open up the chest and stretch the abdominal muscles.

5. Quad Stretch (1 minute per leg): Stretch the front of the thighs.

37

WOD 30

Warm-up:

A light, dynamic warm-up complimenting each movement is recommended. Examples: leg swings, arm circles, torso twists and other dynamic movements to prepare your muscles and joints.

Perform each exercise in order for 3-4 rounds. Rest for 30-60 seconds between each exercise.

Workout:
1. Commando Pull-Ups (8-12 reps)
2. Jump Squats (15 reps)
3. Archer Push-Ups (12 reps)
4. Hanging Leg Raises (15 reps)
5. Handstand Push-Ups (8-10 reps)
6. Muscle-Ups (6 reps)
7. Double Unders (30 reps) or Single Unders (60 reps)

Stretches:

1. Seated Forward Bend (2 minutes): Stretch the hamstrings and lower back.

2. Child's Pose (1 minute): Relax and stretch the lower back, hips, and shoulders.

3. Triceps Stretch (1 minute per arm): Stretch the triceps to relieve tension.

4. Chest Opener Stretch (1 minute): Open up the chest and stretch the shoulders.

5. Quad Stretch (1 minute per leg): Stretch the front of the thighs.

38

Conclusion

CONGRATULATIONS, YOU DID IT! Your body thanks you:) Calisthenics and functionality is a part of your fitness structure now. I hope over these 30 workouts, you've gained not only lean muscle and definition, but a habitual mindset to always better yourself, inside and out. Continue to work hard and stay humble, new and exciting adventures are yet to come! Remember fitness is for everyone, share with friends and family, they'll love it!

If you found this workout guide helpful or life changing in any way, I'd be very appreciative if you left a favorable review on Amazon!

39

References

Active, B. (2022, December 9). Which muscles do calisthenics exercises work? Gravity Fitness Equipment. https://gravity.fitness/blogs/traini ng/which-muscles-do-calisthenics-exercises-work

Planet Fitness. (n.d.). Functional Fitness. Retrieved January 27, 2024, from https://www.planetfitness.com/community/articles/functional-f itness-training

Moldovan, A. (2023, May 9). Crafting a Comprehensive Calisthenics Workout Plan from the Ground Up. Old School Calisthenics. https://o ldschoolcalisthenics.com/calisthenics-workout-plan/

Muscle & Fitness. (2020, August 7). The ultimate functional fitness workout program. Muscle & Fitness. https://www.muscleandfitness.c om/routine/workouts/workout-routines/the-functional-workout-ro utine/

What are Body Mechanics? (n.d.). Jacksonville Orthopaedic Institute. https://www.joionline.net/trending/content/body-mechanics#:~:text

=The%20four%20components%20of%20body,%2Dgroups%2C%20and%20lifting%20technique.

ChatGPT. (n.d.). https://chat.openai.com/

Coles, B. R. (2023, June 7). Legal Disclaimer examples for books. Cascadia Author Services. https://cascadiaauthorservices.com/legal-disclaimer-examples-for-books/#:~:text=If%20you%20engage%20in%20this,action%2C%20known%20or%20unknown%2C%20arising